Time Crunch Fitness & Fast Food

Efficient Workouts and Nutritional Convenience

Table of Contents

Chapter 1. Introduction

In our bustling, time-crunch society, getting fit and eating healthy doesn't have to be a time-consuming affair. Welcome to this Special Report on Time Crunch Fitness & Fast Food: Efficient Workouts and Nutritional Convenience. Seamlessly blending vibrant positivity with practical solutions, this comprehensive guide is designed to help you maximize your well-being without making compromises on your schedule or dietary preferences. We offer intelligent fitness strategies tailored for the modern lifestyle, quick yet savory meals that fuel the body, and indispensable tips on how to efficiently combine both to meet your health goals. Every page promises an enriching journey filled with exciting revelations that will transform your perspective on fitness and nutrition. You won't want to miss out on this game-changing report - it's set to send ripples of change through your life and leave you healthier, happier, and better equipped to tackle your busy schedule.

Chapter 2. Time Crunch Phenomenon: Understanding the Busy Lifestyle

In today's accelerating world, time crunch, also referred to as time poverty, is a pervasive experience not limited to any particular demographic, occupation, or lifestyle. This phenomenon manifests as a relentless scramble against the clock, where every minute seems crammed with tasks and responsibilities.

2.1. The Acceleration of Modern Life

The modern lifestyle could be compared to a speeding vehicle – swift, efficient, and always on the move. In the past, cycles of work and rest often adhered to the rhythms of nature, with ample time dedicated to leisure, community, and reflection. However, with the advent of the Industrial Revolution, our perception and use of time underwent a dramatic shift.

The factory whistle replaced the morning rooster's crow, dictating human schedules with an ironclad regularity that hadn't existed before. As technology advanced and society grew more complex, our lives began to accelerate. The digital revolution of the 21st century accelerated them further, with smartphones and the internet making it possible to work, communicate and consume anytime, from anywhere.

This relentless drive toward productivity and efficiency has led to an oversaturation of our schedules. Work, family commitments, daily errands, self-improvement tasks, social events – the list is endless, and the hours available woefully inadequate.

2.2. Time Scarcity: A Product of our Choices

Despite the technological advancements designed to save us time, the feeling of time scarcity seems more prominent than ever. Why is that so? Social scientists opine that time scarcity is not merely a product of objective conditions but also of the choices we make.

The constant accessibility provided by our digital devices blurs the boundary between work and leisure, causing the former to bleed into the latter. Thanks to smartphones and laptops, our work can follow us into our homes, vacations, and even our beds. Beyond that, social media platforms, designed to harness our attention and time, often rob us of precious hours that could otherwise be used more productively.

Moreover, modern society values busyness and deems it as a mark of status. The busier you are, the more important you seem. Consequently, individuals face implicit pressure to maintain an image of being perpetually occupied. This trend has exacerbated the feeling of time crunch despite there being the same 24 hours in a day that there have always been.

2.3. Impact of Time Crunch on Health and Fitness

The busy lifestyle and ceaseless hustle leave little room for pivotal self-care aspects like sleep, nutrition, and exercise. Due to a lack of time, people often turn to convenient food options that may not be beneficial for their health. Instead of preparing wholesome meals, we habitually resort to quick-fix meals or fast food, contributing to health problems such as obesity, diabetes, and heart disease.

Similarly, our busy schedules often deter us from setting aside time for physical exercise, resulting in long hours of sedentariness. Numerous studies have highlighted the risks associated with chronic inactivity, such as increased susceptibility to weight gain, cardiovascular diseases, and mental health challenges.

2.4. Coping with the Time Crunch

Coping with time crunch doesn't necessarily mean doing more. It involves reassessing and reorganizing our priorities in a manner that accommodates health and wellness. By adopting efficient, tailored strategies, we can nourish our bodies and minds without compromising our productivity.

Firstly, we must bust the myth of multitasking. Studies have shown that multitasking can decrease productivity, as the time loss from switching between tasks often outweighs the perceived efficiency gained. Focusing single-mindedly on tasks helps accomplish them more swiftly and efficiently.

Secondly, it is crucial to establish boundaries, particularly concerning technology. Regular digital detoxes can help preserve personal time undisturbed by work-related or social media disturbances.

Lastly, we should bear in mind that it's okay to say no, recognizing that our time is a finite resource. By declining non-essential activities or requests, more time can be directed towards health and wellness.

2.5. Time Crunch Fitness and Fast Food: A Symmetry

It's vital to understand that a busy lifestyle doesn't mean neglecting health and nutrition – which is where time crunch fitness and fast food come into play. Tailored, efficient workout regimens and quick, healthy meals can seamlessly integrate into the overstuffed modern lifestyle, proving that you can be health-conscious even on a tight schedule.

Efficient workouts don't need to be painstakingly lengthy. High-Intensity Interval Training (HIIT) and other short, intense workouts can offer a complete body workout in a fraction of the time traditional workouts take. Nutritional convenience does not necessarily equate to an unhealthy diet. Fast food can be healthy - it all depends on your choices. Incorporating nutrient-dense quick recipes in your routine such as smoothie bowls, quinoa salads, or roasted veggies can contribute positively to your diet without consuming much time.

A holistic understanding of the time crunch phenomenon and its impact on our lifestyles is the first step towards making positive shifts. By embracing efficiency in both fitness and nutrition, we not only combat the adverse impacts of time scarcity but also achieve a state of balance and wellbeing amidst the hustle of contemporary life.

Chapter 3. Rethink Fitness: Compact, Efficient Workouts for Time-Poor Individuals

In today's fast-paced age, fitting workouts into your schedule might seem like an uphill task. But fear not—the strategies we're about to explore will show you how to maximize your fitness gains while minimizing your commitment to time. Remember, it's about aligning every moment you spend exercising with your overall wellness goal for maximum efficiency.

3.1. Designing Compact Workouts

A significant part of converting your time-strapped lifestyle into a fitness-rich regimen lies in smart workout designs—each meticulously planned to utilize every second, every drop of sweat in achieving your fitness goals. A well-designed compact workout is a potent mix of high-intensity exercises targeting your whole body, focusing on functional movements and multi-joint exercises that engage more muscle groups at once. Examples of such workouts include High-Intensity Interval Training (HIIT), circuit training, supersets, and CrossFit workouts.

HIIT workouts involve periods of maximum-effort exercise followed by short recovery periods. Not only do they maximize calorie burning, but they also significantly improve your aerobic and anaerobic fitness levels.

Similarly, circuit training involves performing a series of exercises in quick succession, providing a full-body workout that burns a high number of calories in a short amount of time.

Supersets push you to perform two exercises back-to-back without a rest period in between. The benefit? Besides saving time, it allows distinct muscle groups to recover while others work—leading to a highly efficient and intense workout.

It's worth mentioning CrossFit workouts. Known for their intensity and versatility, over a limited time, they provide a comprehensive fitness experience covering strength, flexibility, speed, and endurance.

It's essential to understand your fitness level and future objectives. Never jump into an intense regimen without considering your current condition—a balanced, progressive approach is key to any successful workout routine.

3.2. Volume vs. Intensity

When it comes to quick workouts, a common question crops up: should you focus on volume (the total amount of work you do, usually measured in sets and reps) or intensity (how hard you work)?

The answer is simple—intensity. When time is a constraint, efficiency is key, and intensity has been shown to be more effective at spurring fitness improvements than volume. For instance, studies demonstrate that short, intense workouts can yield similar health benefits as longer, lower-intensity workouts.

Moreover, integrating an element of intensity into your workouts can help elevate your metabolic rate post-exercise, often referred to as afterburn effect or Excess Post-Exercise Oxygen Consumption (EPOC). This means you'll continue to burn calories even after finishing your workout—a handy bonus for those seeking weight loss or body toning.

3.3. Effective Time Management of Your Workouts

Time management is the bedrock of compact, efficient workouts. Optimizing your routine to fit your schedule requires strategic planning. Here's how to go about it:

1. Establish time blocks: Jot down all your daily activities and scrutinize where you can slot in quick workout sessions. It could be first thing in the morning, during lunch breaks, or right before bed.

2. Timed workouts: Instead of counting reps, consider timing your exercises. Commit to doing a particular exercise for a set duration—say, 30 seconds or a minute.

3. Active rest period: Instead of complete rest, utilize the rest period to perform low-intensity exercises—this could be yoga stretches or basic calisthenics.

4. Pre-plan your workouts: Knowing what you will be doing before you go into your workout session can cut down on wasted time spent deciding or setting up.

3.4. Bodyweight Exercises for Efficiency

Let's not forget the role bodyweight exercises play in an express fitness routine. They are flexible, require no equipment, and can be done anywhere—your living room, hotel room, or even office! Combined smartly, these exercises can offer both strength training and cardiovascular benefits. The burpee, for example, is an efficient bodyweight exercise that targets multiple muscle groups, gets your heart rate up, and burns plenty of calories.

On a similar note, exercises like push-ups, squats, lunges, sit-ups, jumping jacks, and mountain climbers are versatile and effective bodyweight exercises—you can weave these into an effective routine suited to your strength levels and fitness goals.

3.5. Fitness Technology: Your Ally in Efficiency

Fitness technology today is yet another ally in your quest for compact and efficient workouts. Apps and smart devices can guide you through quick workout routines, track your progress, and remind you to stay consistent. Moreover, they strip away the excuse "I don't know how to do it," as many provide demonstrations and instructions for various exercises.

In conclusion, an efficient workout is more about smart planning than monumental effort. Embrace the techniques of HIIT, circuit training, and supersets. Incorporate bodyweight exercises, leverage fitness technology, and always keep an eye on the clock. Remember, the goal isn't to spend a long time exercising—it's about getting the most out of the time you invest.

Chapter 4. Nutrition Convenience: Fast Food Isn't Always the Enemy

Fast food has carried a troublesome reputation over the years. Too often, it's labeled as the culprit behind an array of health issues, such as obesity, heart disease, and high cholesterol levels. Contrary to this popular tale, however, fast food isn't inherently the enemy. When approached with a savvy mind and a nutrition-focused perspective, it can become an ally in your quest for a healthier lifestyle. Our intention is to educate you on the ways to navigate fast food intelligently without compromising your health, all while making it a convenient aspect of your busy life.

4.1. Demystifying the Fast Food Minefield

Understanding fast food, its components, and its potential impacts is the first step you should take. Nutritionally dense meals can be transformed into the stereotypical harmful fast food thanks to excessive use of unhealthy fats, sugars, and sodium. Being aware of the nutritional value of what you're consuming is key to making better choices. Learn to read and comprehend nutrition fact labels, focusing on calorie count, saturated and trans fat, sodium, and sugar content.

It's important to clarify that not all calories are created equally. The source of these calories - be they from protein, carbs, or fats - plays a significant role as well. A calorie from a sugary soft drink, for example, will not feed your body's needs in the same wholesome way a calorie from a lean, protein-rich chicken breast will.

4.2. Navigating the Menu with Clarity

Making informed choices can become almost second nature if you know what to look out for. Rule of thumb: opt for foods that are grilled, baked, or roasted rather than fried. The method of cooking can drastically modify the nutritional value of a dish. Deep frying, for instance, can hike up the calorie and unhealthy fat content of food.

Portion control is another fundamental aspect. Oversized fast food portions can lead to excessive caloric intake, even with healthier choices. A simple way to navigate this is to opt for smaller sizes, share meals, or save leftovers for later.

Salads, soups, and wraps can be healthier alternatives. However, it's important to check the ingredients that go into them. Beware of hidden calories in dressings, high-sodium broth in soups, and fillings in wraps. Try to spruce up your dishes with fresh veggies to boost dietary fiber, vitamins, and minerals.

4.3. The Drinks Dilemma & Solutions

The drink that accompanies your meal can also heavily impact your caloric intake. Sugar-rich beverages can significantly increase your day's calorie count without contributing much nutritionally. Instead, opt for water, unsweetened tea or even diet sodas if you need a carbonated fix. Be mindful, though, to not make artificially sweetened drinks a daily habit, as they have their own health concerns.

4.4. Fast Food Chains: Continuing to Evolve

Increasing awareness around overall health and wellness is forcing many fast food chains to reconsider their offerings. Numerous popular chains now feature 'lighter' menus with healthier choices. This doesn't mean all their options are healthy, but it does mean you have more potential ways to align your meals with your nutritional needs.

4.5. Creating Customized Orders

Do not hesitate to request modifications for your food to better suit your nutritional needs. Most fast food chains are willing to accommodate these requests. You could consider holding the mayo, choosing a whole-grain bun, or asking for your dressing on the side.

4.6. The Power of Meal Planning and Preparation

The ultimate defense against nutritional compromise is planning. If you have your meals planned and prepared in advance, it's much easier to resist the temptation of unhealthy fast food. Dedicate time each week to plan and cook meals that align with your nutritional goals.

Remember that fast food is not always the enemy. It can be a viable option for a busy schedule, as long as you take the time to understand the nutritional insights it offers. Start by making small changes in your fast food habits and notice the difference over time. Every small, nutritious choice can lead to a lifetime of wellness.

Chapter 5. Breaking the Myth: Fast Food and Healthy Eating Can Coexist

A prevalent misbelief persists in our society - that fast food and healthy eating are polar opposites. The common conception is that fast food, with its cheap prices, convenience and addictive taste, can never lead to good health. However, it doesn't have to be the case. Fast food can indeed be part of a healthy diet with the right knowledge and choices.

5.1. Deconstructing Fast Food

Fast food typically refers to meals prepared and served rapidly, usually within a chain restaurant's framework specializing in such fare. It's often denoted as unhealthy due to a traditionally high concentration of salts, sugars, fats, and overall calorie count.

Nonetheless, we need to understand that not all fast foods are created equal. The nutritional value can fluctuate tremendously based on the ingredients used, the preparation method, the portion size, and the side choices.

5.2. Fast Food Redefined

Change is now upon us, with many establishments undertaking a shift towards healthier renditions of traditional fast food meals. We see fast food chains offering salads, grilled chicken options, low-fat milkshakes, and even whole grain buns. The opportunity is now in the consumer's hands to make better choices amongst a variety of options.

A crucial facet to approach this transformation is learning how to incorporate these alternatives into our diets. Remember, moderation and balance is key. It's not about completely shunning your much-loved burger; it's about substitizing the greasy version with a leaner one and pairing it with a healthy side instead of fried accompaniments.

5.3. Nutrition Labels: Your New Best Friend

Make reading nutrition labels or accessing the restaurant's nutritional information online a habit before ordering. Look for meals low in sugar, salt, and unhealthy fats and high in proteins, fibers, and healthy fats. Additionally, being aware of the calories will help in maintaining a daily dietary balance.

5.4. Portion Control

The size of the serving is an essential factor. Even healthy foods, when eaten in substantial amounts, can contribute to unwanted weight gain. Opting for smaller portions or dividing a larger portion into multiple meals can help manage calorie intake.

5.5. Include More Plant-Based Foods

Vegetables, legumes, and whole grains provide essential nutrients with fewer calories than meat-based options. Look out for options that include these ingredients.

5.6. Mind Your Beverage

Your meal's accompaniments also play a crucial role in your diet. Opt for water or unsweetened iced tea instead of sodas or milkshakes.

Even juices, unless fresh, can be high in sugar and should be consumed sparingly.

5.7. Not All Fats Are Bad

Stay away from trans fats, often found in fried and pre-packaged foods. They increase bad cholesterol and lower good cholesterol, posing significant health risks. Instead, look for sources of healthy fats, such as avocados, nuts, and fish.

5.8. Balancing the Act

Remember when we said moderation and balance are the keys? Don't limit your focus solely on one meal or food. Instead, consider your overall diet. If an unplanned indulgence event happens, balance it with healthier meals throughout the day.

5.9. Don't Fall for Marketing Tricks

Ensure your knowledge trumps tempting advertisements. Just because something is labeled as "low-fat" or "sugar-free" doesn't mean it's necessarily the healthier option. Always check nutritional information to validate the claims.

5.10. The DIY Approach

Lastly, consider making your fast food at home. It may not qualify as 'fast' per se, but investing some time in advance preparation can make the cooking process relatively quick. Plus, you'll have complete control over your meal's ingredients and portion size.

In conclusion, you don't have to sacrifice health for convenience. With education, discipline, and positive choice-making, fast food can indeed coexist with healthy eating in our fast-paced lives. Remember, the power is on your plate!

Chapter 6. Harmonise Fitness and Diet: The Art of Balancing Quick Workouts and Fast Food

Battling the constraints of time in a modern, fast-paced life often culminates in sacrificing either fitness or good nutrition - two components key to our overall well-being. However, achieving delicate equilibrium between these two elements is not merely a stopgap measure, but a sustainable lifestyle modification capable of yielding profound long-term health benefits. This balance allows us to stay fit and eat well, without cannibalizing our time or convenience.

6.1. Ingenious Time-Saving Workout Strategies

Effective fitness routines don't necessarily need to be time-consuming. By tactfully manipulating exercise variables like intensity, frequency, and duration, we can fashion workouts that fit into even the tightest of schedules.

6.1.1. High Intensity Interval Training (HIIT)

HIIT workouts involve alternating short periods of intense anaerobic exercise with less-intense recovery phases. This method significantly cuts down workout duration while ensuring high exertion, making it perfect for the time-poor. A mere 15-30 minutes of HIIT can bring substantial health benefits, from enhancing cardiovascular health to improving metabolism and fat burning.

6.1.2. Circuit Training

This form of body conditioning combines resistance training and high-intensity aerobics, providing a comprehensive workout in just about 20 minutes. By moving promptly through a circuit of 6-10 exercises targeting different muscle groups, with minimal rest between each, you can maximize your workout efficiency and achieve a full-body conditioning.

6.2. Nifty Tricks of the Fast Food Trade

Understanding that fast food doesn't automatically equate to unhealthy food can be life-altering. The trick is to make informed choices that provide the optimal balance of convenience, taste, and nutrition.

6.2.1. Learn to Decode Menus

Cultivating the habit of assessing food not merely on its taste or presentation but also its nutritional content can ease the process of selecting healthy fast food. Look for lean protein sources like grilled chicken, fibers from salads or whole grains, and limit foods that are high in saturated fats, sugars, and sodium.

6.2.2. Consider Portion Sizes

While indulging in fast food, keeping track of portion sizes is crucial to ensure you're not surpassing your daily calorie intake. Choose smaller portions, or split larger meals, to effectively manage caloric intake and keep hunger at bay without piling on unnecessary calories.

6.3. Sure-Fire Ways to Synchronize Fitness and Diet

Once you have a grip on time-efficient workouts and nutritional fast food, the goal is to integrate these two into a synergistic health regimen. Here's how.

6.3.1. Schedule Smartly

Designate regular workout and meal times to streamline your routine. By aligning your food intake with your exercise schedule, you ensure that you fuel and recover adequately, without unnecessary eating.

6.3.2. Listen to Your Body

Every individual's nutritional requirements and fitness capacities are different. Paying attention to how your body responds to different workout routines and meals will enable you to refine your personal balance.

In conclusion, balancing fitness regimes and fast food nutrition might seem daunting in today's high-speed world, but with thought-through strategies, it can become an enjoyable, rewarding, and sustainable lifestyle choice. The path involves carefully selecting workout routines that make the most of every minute and making informed choices while consuming fast food. Finally, the art of harmonizing these elements lies in synchronizing your body's needs with your fitness and dietary routines, setting you on a path towards a healthier, fuller, and more efficient life.

Chapter 7. 5-Minute Meals: Nutritious Recipes for People On the Go

If you're on a tight schedule and it feels like you barely have time to breathe, let alone to prepare a meal, this chapter was written especially for you. With our time-efficient, nutritious, and tasty recipes, you'll discover that you can whip up a healthy feast in as little as five minutes.

7.1. From Your Pantry to Your Plate

One of the keys to quick, healthy meals is a well-stocked pantry. Items like whole grains, canned beans, spices, and frozen vegetables can be the backbone of numerous fast and nutritious dishes.

Here are some pantry essentials that will make your five-minute meals easier:

- Canned legumes: black beans, chickpeas, lentils, and others are protein-rich, versatile, and ready to use.

- Grains such as quinoa, brown rice, bulgur, or whole grain pasta can be cooked ahead of time and stored. This way, they are ready to be added to any dish at a moment's notice.

- Spices: A variety of spices can drastically enhance a meal's flavor, so don't be afraid to load up on things like turmeric, paprika, cumin, and other favorites.

- Frozen vegetables: These veggies are often flash-frozen at peak ripeness, preserving their nutrients and taste. They are great for stir-fries, soups, and other quick meals.

7.2. The Art of Quick Cooking

Every efficient cook knows some techniques or tricks that make their job faster and easier. Here are few tips to remember:

- Use the microwave: Contrary to popular belief, microwaves can be perfectly healthy cooking devices. They're ideal for quickly cooking veggies, defrosting, and reheating leftovers.

- One-pot or one-pan meals: These can save a lot of time by reducing the number of dishes you have to clean afterward. Plus, many one-pot meals require less active cooking time.

- Repurpose leftovers: Incorporating leftovers into new meals can significantly cut down on cooking time, and can result in unique and delicious dishes.

Now that we've covered some ground rules, let's move on to the actual five-minute recipes which will add nutritional magic to your busy schedule.

7.3. Greek Yogurt Parfait

A Greek Yogurt Parfait can be your breakfast, lunch, or dessert. Just remember to prepare your ingredients beforehand for a quicker assembly.

Ingredients: - 1 cup Greek yogurt - 1 cup mixed berries (fresh or thawed out of the freezer) - 2 tablespoons honey - 1/4 cup granola

Procedure: 1. In a glass or bowl, layer half of the Greek yogurt. 2. Add half of the mixed berries and a tablespoon of honey. 3. Add another layer of yogurt, the erstwhile section of the berries, and the remaining honey. 4. Top it off with granola and enjoy!

7.4. Quick Veggie Fried Rice

Leftover rice brings this filling and nutrient-packed meal together in no time. The recipe offers great flexibility, allowing you to use whatever veggies you have on hand.

Ingredients: - 2 cups of cold leftover rice - 1 cup frozen mixed vegetables - 2 tablespoons vegetable oil - 2 eggs - 2 tablespoons low-sodium soy sauce - Optional: sliced scallions, sesame seeds, sriracha

Procedure: 1. Microwave the frozen veggies till they're thawed (typically about 2-3 minutes). 2. While the veggies thaw, heat a large frying pan or wok over medium-high heat. Once hot, add the oil. 3. Crack the eggs into the hot oil and scramble. Once cooked, set them aside. 4. Add the thawed veggies to the pan, stir-fry until heated through. 5. Add the rice and soy sauce to the pan, stirring to combine and break up any big clumps of rice. 6. Add the scrambled eggs back to the pan, stirring again to combine. Serve hot with your favorites toppings.

With these fast and nutritious recipes, you'll have no excuse not to eat healthily, even when the clock is ticking. Remember: eating healthily doesn't need to be a time-consuming ordeal. With a bit of planning, a well-stocked pantry, and a few quick recipes, you'll be well on your way to better eating habits in no time. Enjoy the culinary journey, even in the midst of a time crunch!

Chapter 8. The Importance of Macro and Micro Planning: Scheduling Fitness and Healthy Eating

A successful health journey requires more than ambition. It is circumscribed by structure, order, and attainable goals. By dividing your health ambitions into manageable micro and macro goals, fitness and nutrition become manageable parts of daily life, instead of intimidating monoliths.

8.1. The Macro Perspective

The first step towards optimizing your health is adopting a macro perspective. What are your ultimate goals? Is it to build strength, shed excess weight, cultivate athleticism, or maintain health? This is important to identify because your macro goals influence everything from your exercise routines to nutrition needs.

No fitness journey operates in a vacuum. We all have busy lives, filled with work, family, social, and personal commitments. Scheduling your health within these existing obligations becomes non-negotiable. Have a transparent view of your week. What are essential commitments that cannot be negotiated? These are your immovable objects. Around these, you can strategically schedule your fitness routines and meal timings.

Your fitness should intertwine with your life, not clash with it. A morning jog might work for some, but for those with early morning meetings or late-night shifts, it might be more of an obstacle. Similarly, if you've identified that your energy dips in the afternoons, implementing an afternoon swim or a yoga session could be an energizing boost.

One key takeaway from the macro perspective is having a firm understanding of your overall objectives and properly integrating your fitness journey into your life's existing structure.

8.2. Designing Your Macro Schedule

With your macro goal finalized, it's time to convert it into a workable program. Here's a step-by-step guide.

1. Identify your weekly workout load. How many times a week can you feasibly exercise? This number should be realistic, considering everyday obligations and rest periods.

2. Divide your week into 'Strength', 'Cardio', and 'Rest'. Your macro fitness goal will dictate the proportions.

3. Sync your workouts to your energy levels and commitments. Schedule high-intensity workouts for when you're most energized and low-intensity workouts or rest days for busy days.

4. Use charts or digital calendars. Visualizing your workout schedule can help you manage time effectively and keep motivation high.

8.3. The Micro Perspective

Now, let's apply the same structural principles to our daily schedules to achieve the needed micro perspective. The central pillar of the micro view is timing.

The equation is fairly straightforward. Your body needs fuel to perform a workout, and it also needs nutrients to recover post-workout. Synchronize your meals to your workouts. If you workout in the morning, your breakfast can become a pre-workout meal - fueling you with needed energy. Similarly, your post-workout dinner could be nutrient-rich, aiding in speedy recovery.

Identifying the frequency of your meals (how many times a day will you eat?) and the distribution of your macronutrients (what will you eat and when?) across your day is critical.

8.4. Crafting Your Micro Schedule

Here's a step-by-step guide to develop your micro schedule:

1. Match your meals to your workouts. Have a carb-heavy pre-workout meal for energy and a protein-rich post-workout meal for recovery.

2. Understand your nutrition needs. Your macro fitness goals will dictate your nutrition needs. An aspiring bodybuilder will need more proteins, while someone aiming for cardiovascular endurance will need more carbs.

3. Listen to your body signals. Some of us function well on three large meals a day while others prefer five smaller meals.

4. Use 'MyPlate' or other food-group distribution models to ensure you're getting a proper balance of all the macronutrients.

8.5. Meal Planning & Preparation

Meal planning and preparation is an extension of the micro approach and goes hand in hand with an efficient health journey. It ensures a disciplined approach and helps avoid unplanned eating sprees.

Planning your meals should revolve around your nutritional needs and dietary preferences. This gets much simpler when you know what nutrients you need and when. Preparation can involve batch-cooking or pre-packing meals and snacks.

Planning can be done weekly or bi-weekly, depending on your schedule and fresh food availability. It not only saves time during the week but also ensures consistency in your diet maintaining your nutrition goals.

Conclusively, micro and macro planning of your fitness and healthy eating is a strategic approach. It breaks down the monolithic task of achieving health goals into attainable tasks. It tames the chaos, introduces structure, and seamlessly merges fitness with your life. This not only enhances efficiency but also boosts motivation, keeping you glued to your health journey.

Chapter 9. Transform Fast Food Staples: Healthy Twists on Your Favourite Grab-and-Go Options

Fast food has long been associated with unhealthy eating habits, given the high calorie, fat, and sodium contents commonly found in these meals. However, with some clever substitutions and modifications, it's possible to transform these fast-food staples into healthier alternatives without compromising flavor or convenience.

9.1. Reimagining Burgers

The beloved burger, a fast-food staple, is ripe for healthy innovation. Instead of a classic beef patty, opt for lean proteins like ground turkey, chicken, or even plant-based options. These substitutes slash the saturated-fat count while delivering an ample protein hit.

Further, consider replacing the traditional white bread bun with whole grain alternatives. Whole grains have increased fibre, helping promote feelings of fullness. For an even healthier twist, you can use lettuce or cabbage leaves as a low-carbohydrate, nutrient-dense 'bun.'

Finally, rather than assembling your burger with processed cheese and high-fat sauces, layer in fresh vegetables for added crunch and color. Avocado can provide creaminess, and a homemade sauce such as Greek yogurt with herbs can pack a flavorful punch with fewer calories.

9.2. Enlightening About Fries

Your beloved side of fries need not be a complete no-no. Swap regular potatoes with sweet potatoes, known for their lower glycemic index and higher vitamin content. The real transformation, though, comes via the cooking method. Instead of deep-frying, opt for baking your fries. A drizzle of olive oil, a sprinkle of sea salt, and a hot oven can satisfy your fry cravings with far less fat.

9.3. Rethinking Pizza

The transformation of pizza into a healthier meal involves each of its essential components: the crust, the sauce, the cheese, and the toppings.

First, opt for whole wheat or cauliflower crust over traditional white flour crusts for extra fiber. As for the sauce, bypass store-bought versions high in sugar and sodium. Instead, whip up a quick tomato sauce with fresh tomatoes, garlic, basil, and a hint of olive oil.

Next, practice portion control with cheese, seeking out options with lower sodium and fat content. Finally, rather than topping your pizza with loads of processed meats, opt for a rainbow of vegetables, grilled chicken, or tofu for a protein punch.

9.4. Transforming Tacos

Tacos provide fantastic flexibility for healthy swapping. Start with the tortilla - whole grain or lettuce wraps are healthier alternatives to traditional corn or flour options. Choose lean proteins, like grilled fish or chicken, instead of the more common beef or pork.

As for toppings, pile on veggies instead of excessive cheese and sour cream. Use fresh pico de gallo salsa, avocado, and a drizzle of Greek yoghurt to bring in a burst of colour and flavour without the unhealthy fats.

9.5. Healthy Substitutes for Soda

Hydration is an essential component of any meal, but the calorie count can skyrocket when fast food joints' sugary sodas are involved. For zero empty calories, opt for plain water, herbal tea, or even seltzer water with a splash of fruit juice for flavor.

9.6. The Art of Portion Control

Making healthier substitutes is a crucial step in transforming fast food habits. However, portion control isn't any less important. Most fast food portions far exceed standard serving sizes, leading to inadvertent overeating.

To avoid this, familiarize yourself with standard serving sizes. For instance, a serving of meat should be about the size of your palm. Avoid upsizing meals - even if 'value' meals may seem like a deal, the excessive calories, fats and sugars are anything but valuable for your health.

In conclusion, with some insightful choices and savvy tweaks, your favorite fast food can indeed be part of a healthy, balanced diet. The convenience of quick service meals need not come at the cost of nutrition and well-being. Through the reimagining, enlightening, and transformation of traditional fast food options, we can match the speedy tempo of modern life with a cadence of wellness.

Remember, the road to health is a journey, not a destination. And the goal of this journey is to transform the familiar into an ally of your well-being while retaining enjoyment and convenience. Happy feasting!

Chapter 10. Real-Life Strategies: Stories of Successful Fitness and Nutrition Management

While many of us view fitness and nutrition in terms of scheduled gym hours and carefully calculated meal plans, some folks out there have found a way to integrate these practices naturally into their daily routines. The unsung heroes of modern fitness and nutrition management have made subtle changes to their lives that have yielded impressive results. Join us as we uncover the strategies they deployed to take control of their own health journeys.

10.1. Stepping up with Taylor: Small Changes, Big Progress

Taylor, a busy nurse, proudly embodies the principle that small changes can lead to significant progress. Working 12-hour shifts often meant she was too tired to consider structured workouts or meal planning. Instead of trying to overhaul her routine entirely, Taylor decided to focus on small changes.

She made a promise to herself to take the stairs instead of the elevator at work, encouraged by the dual benefits of added exercise and avoidance of hospital elevators during a pandemic. She also began walking her dog a few blocks further every day. This may sound simple, but moments spent climbing stairs and walking started to add up, and these extra movements eventually triggered a weight loss of 15 pounds over six months.

Nutrition-wise, Taylor asked herself, "What's one habit I can change without feeling deprived?" Her answer was soda. She decided to cut it out and replace it with flavored sparkling water. This simple switch saved her hundreds of calories every week, again contributing significantly to her weight loss journey.

The takeaway from Taylor's story is clear - infusing exercise into your daily routine and making reasonable dietary swaps can lead to significant changes over time.

10.2. Miguel's Magic: Embracing Flexibility

The story of Miguel, a software engineer and father of two, demonstrates the power of flexibility when shaping a fitness and a nutrition regimen. With a demanding job and family responsibilities, Miguel found it impossible to stick to a rigid fitness plan. So he came up with a solution - he decided to break his workouts into multiple mini sessions throughout the day.

Whenever he had a spare 10-15 minutes during a break or on a call, he'd drop down for a round of push-ups, sit-ups, squats, or a quick high-intensity interval training (HIIT) routine without any added equipment. By the end of the day, he'd accumulated a respectable amount of exercise without needing an undisturbed hour at the gym.

One of Miguel's smart nutrition strategies involved the use of a digital nutrition tracker. He quickly found that the process of logging his meals made him more mindful of his portion sizes and the quality of food he was eating. Without feeling restricted in his food choices, Miguel began making healthier choices and losing weight naturally.

Miguel's approach underscores the value in breaking down tasks to fit them into your lifestyle without feeling overwhelmed. Utilizing technology for nutrition tracking also allows greater visibility and control over what goes into your body.

10.3. Gardens and Games with Susan: Making Fitness Fun

For Susan, an architect, fitness had to be enjoyable to have a place in her busy and creative life. Goodbye routines and structures, hello fun! It began with gardening, an activity that she loved and realized could also serve as a form of moderate physical exercise. As she tended to her plants, she'd be carrying bags of soil, climbing ladders, reaching, bending, and squatting - all contributing to her physical fitness.

To enhance her dietary routine, she incorporated more of her garden's fresh produce in her meals, leading to healthier, more nutrient-dense options. Her culinary creativity blossomed along with her garden.

Her second coup was turning family time into fitness time. She planned active games, like tag and frisbee, with her kids. This made fitting in exercise less of a chore and more of an enjoyable family bonding time.

Susan's success inspires us to view fitness as a lifestyle rather than a task, and that incorporating your passions and hobbies into your routine can make the journey enjoyable.

10.4. Sam's Success: Making Meals Meaningful

Sam was a salesman always on the go who relied excessively on fast food. A health scare led him to rethink his nutrition and fitness. Sam started prepping meals during off-hours. He researched and found a plethora of fast, healthy, and easy-to-make meals. He prepped his meals in bulk twice a week, ensuring healthy homemade meals were only a microwave's minute away.

For fitness, he found a 24-hour gym and varied his workout times based on his work schedule. He made a commitment that no matter how busy he was, he'd exercise at least three times a week.

Sam's story calls out to everyone who feels that being on-the-go means a compromise on health. With planning, even the busiest of people can take control of their nutrition. Commitment and flexibility can result in a healthful lifestyle, even within a high-pressure role.

Many of us struggle to fit workouts and planned meals into our packed schedules, often ending up abandoning these routines. The above stories are just a snapshot of the innovative ways that real people are successfully managing to stay fit and eat healthily despite their busy routines. The underlying theme seems to suggest that fitness and nutrition management doesn't necessarily mean adhering to rigid plans. It seems to mean fitting pieces together in a way that suits your lifestyle, interests, and commitments - making the journey more enjoyable and sustainable. Instead of feeling dictated by fitness and nutrition plans, we can choose to sculpt our unique strategies.

Chapter 11. Caring for Your Future: Sustain Healthy Living for a Lifetime

Approaching health as a lifelong journey instead of a short-term objective is crucial in maintaining a vibrant, balanced lifestyle. This approach requires us to shift our focus from temporary changes to sustainable habits. Let's explore strategies, tips, and tweaks to nourish our future and sustain healthy living over a lifetime.

11.1. Building Sustainable Habits

Building sustainable health and fitness habits means integrating exercises and nutritional practices into our routine until they become a natural aspect of our lives. The key to habit building is to start small and gradually increase complexity. Begin with an easier activity, such as a 10-minute walk after dinner each night. As it becomes part of your routine, gradually extend the length of your walks.

It's also essential to choose activities that you enjoy. If you despise running, for example, you're unlikely to perform it in the long-term. Try different activities like dancing, cycling, or yoga until you find one you love.

To manage diet habits, start by adjusting one meal at a time. Enhance breakfast with high-protein foods, add more vegetables to your lunch, or choose wholesome snacks instead of processed ones.

11.2. Creating a Supportive Environment

A conducive environment is crucial in promoting healthy behaviors. Organize your home such that it enhances your wellness objectives: keep workout gear in sight, stock healthy foods in the pantry, and reduce temptation by limiting the presence of unhealthy snacks.

Joining a like-minded community also reinforces your commitment. Local fitness classes or online health forums provide this sense of community and shared goals.

11.3. Mindful Eating

Mindful eating involves paying active attention to the food we consume, savoring each bite instead of mindlessly munching. Pay attention to the texture, flavors, and colors of your food. This practice enhances satiety and enjoyment of meals, reducing the likelihood of overeating.

Start by removing distractions during mealtimes such as television or digital devices. Set a dedicated time slot for meals to focus on food, flavors, and satisfaction cues.

11.4. Regular Health Checkups

Promoting health isn't just about exercise or diet, but also about timely detection and care of any potential health issues. Regular checkups and screenings allow early detection of health issues, effectively keeping them under control.

Identify the types of screenings required based on your age, health history, and lifestyle factors. Keep a regular schedule with your healthcare provider to execute necessary tests.

11.5. Emotional Health and Stress Management

Mental and emotional health plays a substantial role in overall well-being. Stress can hamper wellness efforts and impact physical health. Mitigation strategies can be simple yet highly effective: deep breathing exercises, meditation, spending time with loved ones, or engaging in enjoyable hobbies.

11.6. Sleep: The Fundamental Recovery Tool

Adequate sleep is a pillar of health, profoundly impacting our mood, energy levels, and overall wellness. Create a restful sleep environment free of digital devices and dimly lit. Establish a regular sleep schedule, permitting 7-9 hours of rest each night to allow the body and mind to recover and rejuvenate.

11.7. Modifying Approach With Age

Our body's capabilities change with age, affecting our fitness methodology. Muscle mass and metabolic rate decrease; thus, our exercise program and diet need adaptation.

Include resistance and flexibility training to decrease muscle loss. Adjust daily caloric intake reflecting reduced metabolism, while ensuring nutrient-dense meals persist.

Integrating these lifelong habits allows you to navigate the journey of sustainable health. Remember that perseverance is key. Treat failures as stepping stones, and remember that every decision you make brings you a step closer to your health goals. As you endeavor on this journey, carry forward optimism and an unwavering faith in your capability to create a healthier future.

www.ingramcontent.com/pod-product-compliance
Lightning Source LLC
Chambersburg PA
CBHW060901260726
48661CB00008B/3385